Christian Mental Health

From The Pit Of Fear And Darkness, To Love And Light

JOHN PATRICK

WESTBOW
PRESS®
A DIVISION OF THOMAS NELSON
& ZONDERVAN

WestBow Press books may be ordered through booksellers or by contacting:

WestBow Press
A Division of Thomas Nelson & Zondervan
1663 Liberty Drive
Bloomington, IN 47403
www.westbowpress.com
1 (866) 928-1240

ISBN: 978-1-9736-8233-2 (sc)
ISBN: 978-1-9736-8232-5 (e)

Print information available on the last page.

WestBow Press rev. date: 12/30/2019

Introduction

As a gerontologist who has worked with thousands of adults over the years, and lay minister whose worked in a variety of church ministry roles, it has been a goal of mine to write a few short books about my journey with mental illness, with the hope that they might help facilitate healing in others.

You, the reader, are reading the words from someone who: has been treated unfairly by employers, maintains a home, has struggled financially, has gone without health insurance, has personally experienced mental and physical illness, has had to move their family numerous times, is a spouse, is a father, is a grandparent, and was raised in a highly dysfunctional family. I say this not to seek pity, but to let you know that I'm just like many of you who are reading this book.

After I had finished writing the first draft of this book, I asked myself: *"would someone really be able to easily understand the writings of this book?"* The answer was a definitive no. I felt it was just too theological and philosophical. Some of you will probably feel it's still too theological. I apologize for that. So, I scrapped several hours of writing and re-wrote much of the material in this short book.

I once attended a retreat in WI given by Dr. Gail Brenner, a leading clinical psychologist. I recall Dr. Brenner saying at the retreat: "be careful about not getting permission before giving unsolicited advice." With those words in mind, I wanted to make sure that you, the reader, doesn't feel like all I'm trying to do is give you a bunch of unsolicited advice. I've learned that everyone goes through their own personal healing journey at their own pace and in their own unique way. People receive healing and restoration in a variety of different and individual ways. So, I apologize in advance if you feel I'm giving you unsolicited advice or sound too 'preachy.' It's not my intention whatsoever.

About 15 years ago, I found myself in the deep dark recesses of anxiety and depression. At the time, I truly didn't think I was going to make it *'out of the pit'* as the Psalmist said. I was housebound and was very ill, both mentally and physically. I was totally consumed by fear and it felt like there was no way out. While I did make it out, sadly, my childhood best friend Jack did not.

During my journey to restoration, I learned a variety of 'things' that helped lead me to an improvement in my overall mental health. And the improvement in my mental health, led to an improvement in my physical health, for it's widely accepted that the majority of the physical illnesses that people experience, are mentally or emotionally induced.

I learned it's perfectly okay and actually quite normal to have a mental illness. Most people at some point in their life develop one. I know the National Alliance for Mental Illness (NAMI) is working very hard to eliminate the stigma of mental illness.

I learned and relied on the truth that 'I'm not my own', for scripture says I've been purchased for a price (1Corinthians

6:19-20). So, if I'm not my own and I'm owned by God, then of course God must be causing all things to work together for my good.

The scripture truth that says I'm to *'demolish arguments and every pretension that sets itself up against the knowledge of God, and take captive every thought to make it obedient to Christ'* (2 Corinthians 10:15) was more than just a light bulb going off, it was earth shattering to me.

While no one informed me in advance, I learned that when I decided to become a Christian believer, it was then that the real/hard work actually began. As much as I would have liked to believe and think that God was just going to wipe away and rid me of old, established, habitual fearful patterns of thinking, it didn't work that way for me. I don't think it does for most people either. Wouldn't that be nice if it did?

I learned in my journey about the importance of me doing my part, but just as importantly, to allow God to do God's part.

It's my hope that this short book is just one helpful spiritual aide or tool, in your own healing-journey. If I was removed from 'the pit', average John that I am, I know you will be too, if you've found yourself in one. It's God's promise.

In unity,
John Patrick
Gerontologist
2020

Dedicated to my childhood best friend
Jack, whom we all dearly miss.

Praise the Lord, my soul; all my inmost being, praise his holy name. Praise the Lord, my soul, and forget not all his benefits, who forgives all your sins and heals all your diseases, **who redeems your life from the pit** *and crowns you with love and compassion, who satisfies your desires with good things so that your youth is renewed like the eagle's.*

Psalm 103:1-5

Contents

1

In the beginning

t was a cool, rainy, fall evening. I was on my commute home from work, driving on Interstate 76. Suddenly, out of nowhere, my heart began beating so fast, it felt like it was going to literally jump out of my chest. I immediately exited the freeway at the next exit, pulled up to a convenience store, and called 911. I figured for sure I was having a major heart attack. The paramedics arrived and transported me to the nearest hospital, where I stayed for two days. I underwent several tests, all of which came out negative. I was actually disappointed, for at the time, I would have much rather had an actual diagnosis as to what had caused my heart to beat a million miles a minute. It was an exhausting ordeal. I didn't sleep for several days. What had caused my heart to act this way? I certainly wasn't imagining what I had felt. What if it happened again? What would I do? What if, what if, what if? Over the weeks and months ahead, these constant unexamined 'what if' fears, turned me into an agoraphobic. I became housebound. Just the thought of leaving the house triggered intense physical sensations and emotions. I became too afraid to drive. I felt trapped, like I was in prison being tormented and tortured by fearful spirits.

I had two children at the time, one in college and one in high school. I was the main 'breadwinner'. Would I ever be able to work again? How would I afford my children's college if I couldn't go back to work? Should I apply for disability? Should I admit myself to a psychiatric hospital? Would we have to sell our home? Where would we move to? How would we pay for this or that? I was literally 'in the pit' as the Psalmist said, fearing that there was no way out. This continued on for several months. I lost close to 40 pounds. I knew that if this pace continued, death would be imminent. I began having a variety of physical health problems, that I knew were linked to my inability to properly manage the fear that I had been experiencing. I was experiencing severe GERD (gastro-esophageal reflux disease) because of the tension in my stomach. My stomach acid damaged my vocal cords and throat to the point where I could barely speak and was forced to eat soft food. It was quite a humbling experience going to the grocery store and purchasing baby food for myself. My arms, hands, and fingers were shaking so much, that I was unable to write or print legibly.

One day while listening to Joyce Meyer, she said if we feel too afraid to do something, we need to just get up, get out, and do it anyways. It motivated me to try and drive to work the next day. I recall being about half way to work, when the fearful feelings, emotions, and sensations became so strong and intense, that I ended up turning around and heading back home. While I cried and felt feelings of discouragement, I did see it as sort of a mini-victory, because I did make it half way to work that morning (30 minutes). As I look back, I can clearly remember sitting in my white Chevy Malibu in the plaza's parking lot, fighting with the fear and questioning God. I tried making sense of it all, but was unable to do so. What was I supposed to do next? I just wanted to make it all go away. I did not want my wife and children to know what I was going through. I didn't want them to worry about me or some of the same things that I was worrying about. Little did I know at the time, that fighting and resisting fear, and trying to make it go away or disappear, were not healthy ways to respond to fear. A few days later I did make it to work, only to find myself too afraid to drive home. It was snowing very heavily outside. I remember lying down at work in one of the empty rooms, thinking that it would all just pass. But, it didn't. I didn't know what was wrong with me. I remember calling my wife and asking her if she could pick me up from work. She wasn't very happy with the idea, which was understandable. It was dark outside at the time and the roads were ice and snow covered. It took her nearly two hours to pick me up from work. On the way home, I remember asking her if we should go to the ER. I recall her saying, "John, you've already been down this road before and they found nothing. What makes you think they are going to find something this time?" I have to admit I felt a little angry towards her, thinking that she didn't understand what I was going through.

I ended up staying home from work the next few days. I wasn't sleeping very well, which greatly increased my anxiety levels. I felt too tired and afraid to drive to work. So, one morning, I decided to drive to church. I figured I could make it there since it was only a few miles from home. I recall my body feeling like I had just stuck my finger in an electric receptacle, as I sat in the church pew. My heart was racing and my body was tingling all over.

After the service, I decided to visit the pastor. I recall saying to the Pastor, "Pastor, I feel so afraid and fearful. I don't know what to do about it. I feel like I'm dying." The pastor instructed me to sit down. I sat down and he then prayed over me. I cried and shook, not knowing what to think next. During the short drive home, I remember crying out loud, "God, please help me. I just don't know what else to do." Tears poured down my face. I was thinking that death would actually be much better, than this 'blank' on earth that I was going through.

When I got home, I sat on the couch and turned the TV on. Little did I know, God would hear and answer my cries in the car so quickly. A television commercial came on that asked the question, "Are you suffering from anxiety and depression?" I sat there in silence for a few minutes. I then proceeded upstairs, turned on my computer, and did some research on anxiety. I soon discovered that I, John Patrick, was suffering from GAD (generalized anxiety disorder). I actually felt a sense of relief, now knowing what was causing my mental and physical ailments. But the mental anguish and body discomfort, were as strong as ever.

It was by no means an easy path back to being able to function normally for me. I had become very ill both mentally and physically in just a few short months. There were many moments or times during my period of suffering, where I wondered if I'd ever be able to leave home, travel, or work again.

If you're a Christian believer, and are suffering from anxiety and/or depression, I'm here to give you hope. If I came out of the dark, deep, pit of anxiety, you can and will too. Later on in this book, you'll learn that we can consciously choose to use our 'mind self' to re-focus its 'attention' from fear, to trust in God's Word and promises.

I frequently experienced thoughts such as: I'll never get better, God has abandoned me, or the power of 'the flesh' can't be broken. But I took heed in these encouraging words below taken from the book, *The Cloud of the Unknowing*:

> "Have no fear of the evil one, for he will not dare come near you. Be he ever so cunning, he is powerless to violate the inner sanctuary of your will, although he will sometimes attempt it by indirect means. Even an angel cannot touch your will directly. God alone may enter here."[1]

2

The Soul, flesh, spirit, and mind

*Those who live according to the '**flesh**', set their '**minds**' on what the flesh desires; but those who live in accordance with the '**Spirit**', set their '**minds**' on what the Spirit desires.* (Romans 8:5)

I was able to personally conclude from this scripture passage above, that my **Soul** (*the immaterial essence, animating principle, or actuating cause of my life²*) is accompanied and/or impacted by three different entities, energies, or self's: pick your own word. They are the **flesh,** the **Spirit,** and the **mind**.

The flesh self

Theologians have used many different terms over the centuries to describe the meaning for the word 'flesh' in the Bible. Scripture states that 'the flesh' desires things that are in contrast with what the Holy Spirit desires, and manifests itself by producing thoughts/ inclinations such as: *impurity and debauchery; idolatry; hatred, discord, jealousy, fits of rage, selfish ambition, dissensions, factions and envy; and the like* (Galatians 5:19-21). As scripture says, it's something I strive to deny each day (Matthew 16:23). The word flesh can also be likened to the term concupiscence, as mentioned in the Catechism of the Catholic Church. By the way, I consider myself as a very ecumenical person (*promoting or relating to unity among the world's Christian Churches*). Below is an excerpt from Wikipedia on the word 'concupiscence':

> human nature has not been totally corrupted; rather, human nature has only been weakened and wounded, subject to ignorance, suffering, the domination of death, and the inclination to sin and evil (CCC 405, 418). This inclination toward sin and evil is called 'concupiscence' (CCC 405, 418). Baptism, CCC teaches, erases original sin and turns a man back towards God. The inclination toward sin and evil persists, however, and he must continue to struggle against concupiscence (CCC 2520).[3]

The Spirit self

*But the Advocate, the Holy Spirit, whom the Father will send in my name, will teach you all things and will **remind** you of everything I have said to you* (John 14:26).

I am the temple of the Holy Spirit (1 Corinthians 6:19-20). God living and dwelling in me. I had read this scripture verse many times before, but it never fully resonated with me until I found myself in the deep, dark pit of fear. Scripture refers to the Holy Spirit as the Spirit of Truth (John 16:13). Back in Jesus' days, they didn't have Bibles to pass around. So, the Holy Spirit's presence was needed to help *'remind'* Christian believers of the Word that they heard. Today, we are fortunate to have the Holy Spirit, the Spirit of Truth, in written Word.

Scripture says the 'Spirit' self manifests itself as: *love, joy, peace, forbearance, kindness, goodness, faithfulness, gentleness and self-control* (Galatians 5:22).

The mind self

Until I was enlightened by God's Word, I never fully understood what the **mind** self's purpose and function was. God has uniquely gifted me with a 'mind'. As Romans 8:5 says above, the 'mind self' **sets its attention** on thoughts of the **flesh** *(i.e. falsities such as fear, anger, envy, guilt, want, etc.)* or on thoughts of the **Spirit** *(i.e. truths such as love, joy, peace, patience, kindness, etc.)*. As will be discussed in greater detail later in this book, Romans 8:5 basically implies that 'thoughts', and the 'mind', are two totally separate and distinct entities. Remember this life-changing and healing truth.

3

The Holy Spirit

But when He, the Spirit of truth comes, he will
guide *you into all the truth.* (John 16:13)

W hen I (Soul) was baptized with the Holy Spirit, I became a new man. A new creation in Christ.

Therefore, if anyone is in Christ, the new creation has come. The old has gone the new is here (2 Corinthians 5:17)

The Holy Spirit, the Spirit of Truth, would one day help ***guide*** me with my *holding thoughts captive for truthfulness* activity that scripture commands. I learned that this 'belt of truth' buckled around my waist (Ephesians 6:14), was a key 'piece of armor' (Ephesians 6:11) that I needed, in order to ensure I, 'mind self', **set its attention** on things of the Spirit (Philippians 4:8), rather than on things of the flesh (Romans 8:5).

Ever wonder if you've received the Holy Spirit, the Spirit of Truth? I know I did. Here are some words from Rev. Richard Rohr that I found very helpful:

"To be filled with the Spirit, we must ask for the Spirit. But it is not enough to ask with our lips. We have to empty ourselves of our self-sufficiency if we are to receive the Holy Spirit. We have to empty ourselves of all our idols, if we are to have room for the true God within us. We have to be like the Apostles in the upper room, aware of our nothingness, so that God the creator can make something happen out of nothing. To experience the Spirit, we must yearn for the Spirit. We must seek it, desire it, long for it. We must make ourselves ready to receive God's gift by asking for it not only with our mind but also with our heart and with our gut. Jesus said, "Ask and you will receive," but if we do not really ask, how can we ever truly receive? When we have done all that, all we can do is let God love us, let God give grace to us, let God be gracious to us, let God shower gifts on us. If we wait in patient expectation, the Lord will come. If we do not try to be worthy, the Spirit will be given. If we trust in God's promise, we will not be disappointed. Any way it happens is just as real, just as good as any other. The Lord meets us where we are, and he makes his presence known to us in the way we are most ready to experience it. God can only fill the emptiness we bring to him, but if we ask the Lord to fill it, we cannot be disappointed. The Spirit cannot withhold itself from any heart that longs to know the powerful presence of God. When it does happen, we know we did nothing to deserve it. We realize it's pure gift."[4]

I/mind self's decision to confess with my mouth and believe in my heart that Jesus was Lord, and asking for the Holy Spirit to be poured out into my heart, made me a temple of the living God (1 Corinthians 6:19).

If you aren't sure if you've ever received the Holy Spirit, I encourage you to speak with your church. I'm sure they would be glad to assist you.

4

Hold that thought - renewing the mind

*We demolish arguments and every pretension that sets
itself up against the knowledge of God, and **we take
captive every thought** to make it obedient to Christ*
(2 Corinthians 10:5)

While sitting on the couch one day reading this scripture verse above, it seemed to me that God was saying:

*John, since I instructed you through my Word to use
your '**mind self**' that I gave you, to hold thoughts
captive, make them obedient to my word, and set
its attention on whatever is true (Philippians 4:8),
this means **thoughts are totally and completely
meaningless and irrelevant**. YOU ARE NOT
THOUGHTS, you're MIND, as well as Soul and
Spirit.*

WOW! I actually felt a little stunned and shocked. Did I really hear and understand this correctly?

I am NOT thoughts? Seriously?

I had spent years fretting about, arguing with, worrying about, trying to change, or rid myself of fearful thoughts, and now you're telling me God that thoughts are not me, and are therefore completely meaningless?

This was the beginning of my healing journey

2 Corinthians 10:5 instructed me that I'm not to simply sit still idly by and allow unhealthy fearful or worrisome thoughts to just continue on with free rein. I'm to use my 'mind self' to make a conscious-willful decision or choice, to use ALL THREE of its God given **'mind'** functions and abilities, in regards to thoughts. Think of the letters AAA.

1) AWARE of what they're saying
2) ASSESS for truthfulness (*hold them captive*)
3) Set/move ATTENTION to the Truth, g-e-n-t-l-y, if a false one is noticed/discovered in #2.

Here's an example as to how it works. In the past, I'd experience a fearful thought such as '*what if*' I lost my job or became unable to work. For me, those were big fears. The fears would often produce real, intense, emotions that caused a variety of very uncomfortable physical sensations throughout my body. What did I used to do? I would try different things to ignore, resist, suppress, or eliminate the fearful thoughts and/or feelings. This just strengthened and intensified them, for as the great Swiss psychologist Carl Jung once said, "*whatever we resist, persists.*" My 'mind self' completed and stopped at step one (*was **aware** of the fearful thought and what is was saying*), but didn't use its full capabilities. It skipped step 2 *(assess/hold thought captive for truth),* therefore maintaining its (set) **attention** on the fearful thought. Over time, my 'mind self's' continual, perpetual, **set attention** on the fear, made it grow stronger and stronger, until it became a stronghold and began causing mental and physical dis-ease.

Today, I handle this situation much differently. What I do now, is use the full power of my '**mind self**' that God gave me:

- I'm **AWARE** of the unhealthy fearful thought (*what if I lose my job?*)
- I **ASSESS** it for truthfulness per God's Word. (*It's false, because God's Word says He will provide for all my needs according to His glorious riches - Philippians 4:8*)
- I set/move its **ATTENTION** to this truth

I learned the liberating Truth from 2 Corinthians 10:5 that I'm not thoughts, I'm 'mind self' who: is aware of thoughts, assesses thoughts, and sets its attention on Truth. The fighting with, denying, worrying about, suppressing, and trying to change or eliminate fearful thinking stopped. They truly are meaningless & irrelevant. I began to befriend them, welcome them, and actually become comfortable with their presence and existence.

I reflected for several weeks on this new conviction or revelation, testing it, examining it, and analyzing it for Truth. Could this really be that 'igniting' of the Holy Spirit that I so desperately longed for, to *redeem my life from the pit and crown it with love and compassion* (Psalm 103:4)? Could this be the beginning of my healing and restoration from my slavery and captivity to fear, worry, and agoraphobia? I felt a new encouragement that I hadn't felt in a long time.

> *For the word of God is alive and active. Sharper than any double-edged sword, it penetrates even to dividing soul and spirit, joints and marrow; it **judges the thoughts** and attitudes of the heart.* (Hebrews 4:12)

The Word of God is used to judge the thoughts and attitudes of the heart. BINGO! This scripture reaffirmed that I was on the right track and headed in the right direction: gently engaging 'mind self' to recognize and confront **'normal'** thought falsities and lies with Truth. You might be thinking: *"I can't do this." "It hurts too much." "It's too painful." "I don't have the stamina or energy to do it."* Yes, it is difficult in the beginning. Yes, there is pain. But I learned that pain was totally normal and was actually a good sign. An inner purification process was going on inside of me, with God's Word being the facilitator and healer. The Truth was setting me free. Slowly but surely, stored up lies, fears, and anxieties from the past began releasing themselves. As a matter of fact, my body experienced MORE anxiety at first, when I used ALL the capabilities of my 'mind self' to confront unhealthy fearful thinking with Truth. Because, the 'thought producing mechanisms' were just used to, or in the habit of, doing whatever they wanted and having 'free-rein'. To this day, I still heavily rely on this scripture truth below, when I experience thoughts of doubt, as to whether or not I can be victorious over fear or the power of evil:

> *You, dear children, are from God and have overcome them, because the one who is in you is greater than the one who is in the world. (1 John 4:4).*

I knew, I just knew that with God's grace, Truth, and presence within me through the Holy Spirit, I could persevere, endure, and be set free from the dominion of fear. Because, *I can do all this through him who gives me strength.* (Philippians 4:13).

Since God's Word says I'm being t-r-a-n-s-f-o-r-m-e-d by the renewal of my mind (Romans 12:2), of course that meant it would take time for me to experience healing and renewal.

This may sound very odd and strange to you right now if you're in the pit, but, in time it will 'sink-in'. With my 'mind self', I actually began choosing to rejoice and be glad when my 'mind self' noticed unhealthy fearful thoughts, feelings, or emotions. Why? Well, listen to God's Word:

> *But he said to me, "My grace is sufficient for you, for my power is made perfect in weakness." Therefore I will boast all the more gladly about my weaknesses, so that Christ's power may rest on me. That is why, for Christ's sake, I delight in weaknesses, in insults, in hardships, in persecutions, in difficulties. For when I am weak, then I am strong. (2 Corinthians 12:9-11).*

That's a pretty powerful Truth. Unhealthy fearful thoughts still occur, but with much less frequency and intensity. It all started to begin making sense. For years I hadn't held thoughts captive for truthfulness. This meant that all along, I was automatically and unconsciously discerning all thoughts to be true. I must admit in the beginning of my healing journey, I experienced thoughts such as: *"God, seriously, why do things have to be this way? Why don't you just 'wipe away' the remaining influence of the flesh/old man self* (Ephesians 4:22) *when I became a Christian? Why make me have to go through all this effort of holding thoughts captive for truthfulness?"* I concluded that it wasn't worth the time or energy to try to figure this question out. Since no human being has ever come up with the answer, what would make me think that I could?

You may be thinking: *John are you serious? Do you really expect me to 'hold thoughts captive' all the time?* I know, I felt the same way at first. At first it did seem a little overwhelming. But like any good cognitive behavioral therapy practice or technique, it requires some personal effort. But the good news is, for almost all of the unhealthy/negative thoughts that my 'mind self' holds captive, my 'mind self' can gently use one short **'proclamation'** of Truth taken from the Gospel of Matthew Chapter 6:

> *I (Soul, mind, and Spirit)* **don't worry about my life, body, or tomorrow.**

I encourage you to memorize these 13 words. They will be your 'belt of truth' and 'armor' throughout your entire life, bringing you comfort, consolation, and rest to your soul.

Jesus did say that in this world I would experience trouble and suffering. But He also says I'm to take heart, for He has overcome the world (John 16:33). I had often wondered what Jesus meant by this passage. I believe the Book of Romans provides the answer:

> *Not only so, but we also glory in our sufferings, because we know that suffering produces perseverance; perseverance, character; and character, hope. And hope does not put us to shame, because God's love has been poured out into our hearts through the Holy Spirit, who has been given to us.* (Romans 5:3-5)

I held firm to Jesus' words: *you will know the truth, and the Truth WILL set you free* (John 8:32). Free from my being's slavery to, and power of, unhealthy, perpetual, unceasing, constant fearful thinking. I held firm that if I endured and persevered in my 'mind renewal' journey, I would eventually like the Apostle Paul, learn the *secret to being content in ALL circumstances* (Philippians 4:12). Isn't that an amazing scripture truth and promise, learning to be content in all circumstances? The good news is, we are all on our way to that state.

William James, often referred to as the father of American psychology, once said:

> "The greatest weapon against stress, is our ability to choose one thought over another."

This directly applied to what I learned I was called to do as a Christian believer with my 'mind self': to hold thoughts captive for truthfulness. But what about at night? What about when I'm lying in bed trying to fall asleep? I'd be up all night if I engaged my mind in holding thoughts captive. Well, I have some very good news for you. Since I/mind self consciously chooses to 'take a break' from all *'hold thought captive'* activity while lying in bed, this means that all thoughts that I experience while lying in bed, are totally 100% meaningless. WHEW! That being said, what am I supposed to do with my 'mind self' attention while lying in bed, if it's not actively involved in holding thoughts captive? It's moved to the present moment through use of the senses. Such as: this bed **feels** great or I **hear** my calm relaxed breathing. Not much to see, taste, or smell at this time.

During some of my past one hour commutes to work, I frequently listened to Christian radio programming. This activity helped me with my renewal of my mind journey. The benefit? Less encountering of negative thoughts and more noticing of positive thoughts. Most areas of the country now have a Christian radio station, be it K-LOVE, Moody Radio, or another local Christian radio station or network. I can't help but thank Moody radio for their radio ministry. Listening to Chuck Swindoll's Insight for Living, The Alternative with Dr. Tony Evans, and Joni and Friends with Joni Eareckson Tada, were all instrumental in my recovery. Thank you Moody radio for your ministry. You are much appreciated and valued.

5

Prayer

Meditative prayer

Meditative prayer can be described as the deliberate/conscious use of one's mind self, to engage in some spiritual or religious activity. It's a 'doing' more than a 'being'. It can involve activities such as: reading books, saying prayers, listening to messages or music, or physically engaging in some other spiritual or religious activity.

By engaging in balanced/moderate meditative prayer, I did notice a reduction in the number and severity of anxious and fearful thoughts. Besides regular reading and listening to music, I found two ministries that were especially helpful to me with my meditative prayer. First, is the Worldwide Community for Christian Meditation www.wccm.org It was founded by John Main in 1975. Second, is The Christian Meditator website, www.thechristianmeditator.com, founded by Rhonda Jones. Rhonda has an outstanding selection of Christian audio meditations, which greatly helped me with my renewal of my mind journey. I highly recommend her resources.

Christian contemplative prayer

Come to me, all you who are weary and burdened,
and I will give you rest. (Matthew 11:28)

Be still and know that I am God. (Psalm 46:10)

At some point, I began finding it a real struggle to engage in meditative spiritual practices and activities. And, I did not see any difference or reduction in the frequency or intensity of the fears that I was experiencing. So, being the achiever/type 3 that I am (Enneagram), I worked harder and harder on my meditative prayer. I prayed more often, read more spiritual books, and attended religious services more frequently. The result? I became even <u>more</u> anxious. Then thankfully by God's grace, and God ALWAYS came through when it felt like I was at the end of my rope, I came across the classic writings of St. John of the Cross's '*Dark Night of the Soul*'. St. John wrote about the time in some Christian believers' lives, where God calls them to move away from a meditative prayer life, and towards a more contemplative prayer life: spending time in stillness, silence, and solitude in God's presence. I sensed in my being that God was calling me to take a rest or break from my meditative prayer pursuits and activities. I had worked myself to exhaustion, trying to eliminate fearful and anxious thoughts and feelings. But as St. John of the Cross states below, engaging in 'more' spiritual activities, can actually make things worse like it did for me.

Below was, and still is, a very powerful and transforming teaching for me. It's from Chapter 10 of St. John of the Cross's 'Dark Night of the Soul' writing. I encourage you to read it slowly and carefully, so you get the message.

Chapter 10

Of the way in which souls are to conduct themselves in the dark night.

DURING the time, then, of the aridities of this night of sense wherein it no longer has any power to work or to reason with its faculties concerning the things of God, as has been said, spiritual persons suffer great trials, by reason not so much of the aridities which they suffer, as of the fear which they have of being lost on the road, thinking that all spiritual blessing is over for them and that God has abandoned them, since they find no help or pleasure in good things. Then they grow weary, and endeavor (as they have been accustomed to do) to concentrate their faculties with some degree of pleasure upon some object of meditation, thinking that, when they are not doing this, they are doing nothing. This effort they make brings great inward repugnance on their soul, which was taking pleasure in being in that quietness and ease, instead of working with its faculties. These souls turn back at such a time if there is no one who understands them; they abandon the road or lose courage. Thus, they fatigue and overwork their nature, imagining that they are failing through negligence or sin. Let them trust in God, who abandons not those that seek Him with a simple and right heart, and will not fail to give them what is needful for the road, until He bring them into the clear and pure light of love. The way in which they are to conduct themselves in this night of sense is to devote themselves <u>not at all to reasoning, since this is not the time for it, but to allow the soul to remain in peace and quietness</u>, although it may seem clear to them that they are doing nothing and are wasting their time, and although it may appear to them that it is because of their weakness that they have no desire in that state to think of anything. The truth is that they will be doing quite sufficient if they have patience and persevere in prayer without making any effort. What they must do is merely to leave the soul free and disencumbered and at rest from all knowledge and thought, troubling not themselves about what they shall think or meditate upon, but contenting themselves with merely a peaceful and loving attentiveness toward God, and in being without anxiety, without the ability and without desired to have experience of Him or to perceive Him. And although further scruples may come to them—that they are wasting their time, and that it would be well for them to do something else, because they can neither do nor think anything in prayer— let them suffer these scruples and remain in peace, as there is no question save of their being at ease and having freedom of spirit. [5]

As previously stated, this was a very enlightening and transformative teaching for me. It taught me the importance of taking regular time to be still in God's presence and rest my faculties. Not doing or expecting anything. Just resting in God's presence, knowing God was doing the doing (*restoring*), and I was doing the being (*receiving*). The timing couldn't have been better, for I was working myself sick, trying to be more spiritual and religious, in order to make the fears and anxieties just go away.

Lucinda Bassett, renowned author, speaker, and founder of the Midwest Center for Stress and Anxiety, once experienced debilitating anxiety and depression herself. I once heard her speak about the importance of spending time each morning in stillness and quiet, before she began her day. I think of the incredibly gifted author, teacher, and speaker Joyce Meyer. I remember listening to Joyce on the radio one time say that when she woke up in the morning, she strived to spend the first part of her day in silence and quiet.

For me, in order to receive the full healing/restorative power of God, to attain the inner peace and restoration that I so strongly desired, God was calling me to spend regular time with Him in silence, solitude, and stillness. Ideally, twice a day, for at least 20 minutes at a time.

If you find yourself feeling like I did, struggling with regular meditative prayer activities, God may be calling you to a new form of prayer; Christian contemplative prayer.

For teaching and instruction on Christian contemplative prayer, I recommend the 'Contemplative Outreach' organization founded by Rev. Thomas Keating. Rev. Keating wrote an excellent book called *Open Mind Open Heart,* on the meaning and practice of contemplative/centering prayer. Rev. Keating points out in his book, and I can attest to every one of them, that contemplative/centering prayer can produce many wonderful healing and restorative benefits: 1) it calms the mind, 2) it calms the affective nervous system, 3) it gives one more energy, and 4) it helps one experience God's presence more deeply. How about those benefits? If someone told me I could partake in a free activity that produced these benefits, I'd immediately want to know more.

According to one of the first books ever written on the subject of Christian contemplative prayer, *The Cloud of the Unknowing*, the book's authors reference two other powerful benefits of contemplative prayer: improvement in one's sleep and the complete healing from the desires of the flesh. Wow! I can't say I've attained complete healing from the flesh, but, I can say that my mind is a lot better at managing the desires of the flesh than it used to be. Just think what the world would be like if everyone engaged in contemplative prayer and received healing from the desires of the flesh. What a peaceful world we'd live in.

The Contemplative Outreach organization has produced a short educational video on the topic of centering/contemplative prayer. You can find it on YouTube at the following web address: www.youtube.com/watch?v=AZ3s9Stgt80. I've had the privilege of personally meeting Mary Dwyer, the instructor in the video. She is a very gifted individual. This form of prayer is actually very ecumenical. I've met people from various denominations and religious backgrounds, who practice this early church practice of contemplative prayer. I encourage you to visit the Contemplative Outreach website, to see if there are any centering prayer groups in your area that you can learn from and possibly participate in, if you feel called to do so. I've participated in contemplative prayer groups in Ohio, North Carolina, Georgia, and Florida. I am by no means a devout contemplative prayer practitioner. But, had I not learned about this early church practice during my dark time of anxiety and depression, I might still be stuck in the pit.

Prayer for healing ministries

What about prayer for healing ministries? I do have some personal experience in this area. When I was in my 20's, I experienced major low back pain. I went to numerous doctors and had tried a variety of self-help remedies and techniques. Nothing worked. Then, one night, I noticed that the church I attended was having a prayer for healing service. During the service, the woman who was leading the service said someone in the back of the church was being healed from a back injury. I happened to be sitting in the last row. I began feeling an intense/radiating heat in my lower back. The usher nearby noticed me and escorted me up to the front of the church. The healing minister and Pastor laid hands on me and I went down. Everyone was praying and singing. If there is a heaven on earth, that time spent lying on the altar floor was it. It was simply beautiful. The next day when I woke up, I noticed my back pain was gone and it never came back. It truly was and still is a mystery. Why did God choose to heal me that Saturday evening? I have no idea. Perhaps he wanted me to someday write a series of short books on the subject of Christian Mental Health, like I'm presently doing now. So, when someone asks me if they should attend a prayer for healing service, my response is, "sure, why not?" Even if the person is not healed from the specific condition that they were hoping they would receive healing for, based on my experience in healing ministry, I believe

God DOES heal them in some unique, unknown, and special way. As far as places that one can go to in Florida for healing prayer, I highly recommend Christian Healing Ministries in Jacksonville (founded by Francis and Judith MacNutt), and The Inheritance House in Orlando. Both of these wonderful healing ministries are solid in their missions, visions, and purposes.

Christian prayer for healing

The following is a prayer for healing based entirely on scripture truth, that I composed a few years ago.

> God the Father, Son, and Holy Spirit, my 'mind self' consents to your presence and action within me. You tell me to bring my prayer requests to you with a spirit of thanksgiving, and then your peace, which surpasses all understanding, will guard my heart and mind in you. Since you mysteriously cause all things to work together for my good, I choose to trust you, and not to believe the 'old man self's' constant desire to want to know why things have, or are, happening the way they are. I proclaim, like Mary, "Your will be done." And since it is being done, my 'mind self' chooses to give thanks in all circumstances. I know that sometimes, like in the Book of Genesis with Joseph, I may be a recipient of evil, and yet somehow, some way, you're able to bring good out of it. I choose to walk by 'faith' in

you, and not by what I 'see' happening around me. Help me to manifest your 'fruits' in my thoughts, words and actions. It's very healing and liberating for me as a Christian to know, that as a Christian, my thoughts and feelings are totally meaningless, until I first make the conscious effort to assess them for truthfulness according to Your Word, and g-e-n-t-l-y refute those that are not, with your Truth. I know the 'flesh/old man' self loves to conjure up thoughts and feelings of fear and worry. However, my 'new man/spirit' self, part of my REAL identity, doesn't worry about my life, body, or tomorrow, for you're providing for all my needs according to your glorious riches. Continue to help me in my 'transformation by the renewal of my mind' journey. Thank you for the truth that **there is nothing that can ever separate me from your love and mercy.** As the purchaser of my being, thank you for taking all the 'normal' cares and anxieties of the 'flesh/old man' self. When I come to you in stillness, silence, and solitude, you give me rest. I know that when I experience a 'thorn in the flesh', your grace is sufficient for me, for your power is being made perfect in me. You never allow me to be tempted beyond my ability to resist, for I can do all things THROUGH YOU, who gives me the power. After I've suffered a little while, you will restore me and make me strong, firm, and steadfast. Like the Apostle Paul, I know that when my body does things that I did not want it to do, it wasn't the real 'me, 'new/man/spirit' self that did it, it was the 'flesh/old man' self that did it. So, I'm never condemned by you. However, your Word says that I'm not to use this new freedom as an excuse to satisfy the desires of the 'old' self, but I'm to strive to serve one another in love. Since you'll never leave or forsake me, I say with confidence, you're my helper, I'm not afraid, there is nothing man can do to me. You're my Shepherd, I do not want. Greater are you that who lives within me, than he that who lives in the world. Thank you for your Word, **that has set me free.**

A prayer of surrender

The following is an anonymous prayer of surrender to God, that I think does an excellent job of reminding us about the importance of making a daily/conscious decision to trust in God's presence and action within us, and the importance of continuously casting the cares of the 'flesh/old man self' upon the Lord:

Why get agitated? Let me take care of all your business. I shall be the one who will think about them. I am waiting for nothing else than your surrender to me, and then you do not have to worry any more about anything. Say farewell to all fears and discouragement. You demonstrate that you do not trust me. On the contrary, you must rely blindly on me. To surrender means: to turn your thoughts away from troubles, to turn them away from difficulties you encounter, and from all your problems. Leave everything into my hands, saying, "Lord, Thy will be done. Thou think of it." That is to say: "Lord, I thank you, for you have taken everything in your hands, and you will resolve this for my highest good." Remember that thinking of the consequences of a thing is contrary to surrender. That is to say, when you worry that a situation has not had the desired outcome, you thus demonstrate that you do not believe in my love for you. You will prove that you do not consider your life to be under my control and that nothing escapes me. Never think: How is this to end? What is going to happen? If you give into this temptation, you demonstrate that you do not trust me. Do you want me to deal with it...yes or no? Then you must stop being anxious about it! I shall guide you only if you completely surrender to me and when I must lead you into on a different path than the one that you expect, I carry you in my arms. What seriously upsets you is your reasoning, your worrying, your obsession, your will to provide for yourselves at any price. I can do so many things when the being, as much in his material necessities as in his spiritual ones, turns to Me saying: "You think of it." Then, he closes his eyes and rests quietly. You will receive a lot but only when your prayer relies fully upon Me. You pray to me when in pain so that I intervene, but in the way you desire it. You do not rely on me, but you want me to adjust your requests. Don't behave like sick ones who ask a treatment of the doctor, all the time suggesting it to him. Do not do that; but rather, even in sad circumstances, say: "Lord I praise and thank You for this problem, for this necessity. I pray you to arrange things as you please for this terrestrial and temporal life. You know very well what is best for me." Sometimes you feel that disasters increase instead of diminish. Do not get agitated. Close your eyes and tell me with faith: "Thy will be done. You think of it." And when you speak thus, I accomplish a miracle when necessary. I only think of it when you trust me totally. I always think of you, but I can only help you completely when you rely fully on me.

6

The emotion of fear

F earful emotions are very real and can be quite intense. Fear often triggers the adrenal glands to secrete hormones into the bloodstream that cause noticeable physiological responses *(rapid heart rate, tingling, sweats, chills, lump in the throat, mental confusion, weakness in the limbs, and so on)*. These symptoms used to come on so quickly and forcefully, I often could barely think or function straight. I had never received the proper tools or training on how to effectively deal with fear and fearful emotions when they occurred. As anthropologists tell us, fear and judgmental thinking are just wired in our circuits. They are more powerful than reason and are the root cause of many mental health issues.

I experienced thoughts such as: *John, if you were doing it right, you wouldn't continue to have thoughts or feelings of fear, because, after all, doesn't scripture say in numerous places, BE NOT AFRAID?* However, I came to the conclusion that what this scripture actually implied, was that I wasn't to remain afraid, with my mind self's attention remaining 'set' on the fearful thinking.

I personally recommend the writings and teachings of noted author and clinical psychologist Dr. Gail Brenner. Dr. Brenner has a host of excellent resources available on her website, on how we can effectively deal with emotions, especially fear, in healthy ways. You can visit Dr. Brenner's website at: www.gailbrenner.com Here is a link to one of her videos titled 'Lovingly being with fear': https://www.youtube.com/watch?v=8wtscQLkjfU

I regularly recommend her guided audio meditations that are available for purchase on her website. I believe they are one of the best investments a person can make, if they are serious about their self-care and overall health and well-being. As a matter of fact, I tell people if they can commit to listening to Dr. Brenner's first audio in Volume 1, titled *Ease and Relaxation*, once after waking up and once before going to bed, they will notice a greater sense of peace in a very short time. Who wouldn't desire more of that?

When a normal, unhealthy, strong fearful feeling or emotion pops up, we've found the following action steps may be helpful:

- Take three long/deep breaths (*this relaxes the central nervous system*).
- Acknowledge, accept, and welcome the totally normal fear from the 'old man/flesh'. Smile!
- Re-focus the mind's **attention** away from any negative stories or commentaries going on in the brain, to the physical sensations in the body
- Proclaim the truth: *I don't worry about my life, body, or tomorrow, because God owns me and is causing all things to work together for my good.*

- Move the mind's attention/focus to the here and now (*present moment*): what is seen, heard, smelled, tasted, or touched.
- Thank God for the experience, knowing God's power is being perfected in us.
- Give/cast the fear to God

As mentioned previously in this book, I went through a phase of believing that if I was just more spiritual or holy, I would no longer experience fearful thoughts, feelings, or emotions. I eventually learned that that was another lie initiated from the remnants of the 'flesh/old man' self. Every human being has experienced, and will continue to experience, episodes of fear. I'll not be completely set free from the remnants of the 'flesh/old man' self, until my Soul leaves my physical/earthly body and is fully united with God.

The key point that I remind myself of many times each day, is since I, 'mind self', is instructed in God's Word to hold thoughts captive, that means **thoughts** (*regardless of how or where they come from*) **aren't me. They're totally meaningless and irrelevant. What healing, liberating, restoring truth!**

Here's some additional advice from a blog written by Dr. Gail Brenner, on dealing with emotions in a healthy manner:

> Your attempts to change them fail, so you feel resigned to feeling that way forever. If these sound familiar to you, then your way of dealing with emotions isn't working. These strategies keep you hooked. Can you see yourself in any of these? If you

move toward emotions, you indulge them. They are so important. You build elaborate stories around them that are all-encompassing and dramatic. You think and talk about them with great relish. You might say some version of, "I'm so upset! Can you believe he did that?" Moving toward emotions keeps them very much alive in you with no chance for relief. If you move against emotions, you fight them. You hate how you feel. Your attempts to control these feelings don't work, but you are at a loss as to what to do about them. Before you know it, you've said hurtful words. Even your body may feel like it's on fire. People who move against often feel anger and frustration. You may even justify how you feel, which keeps the feeling firmly locked in place. Moving away from emotions may be the most common reaction. You avoid them like the plague. Instead of experiencing what is present, you eat or drink to excess, stay too busy, and get stuck in endless thinking. Anything so that you don't have to feel them. An ignored emotion stays hidden, and a hidden emotion is an invitation for inadequacy, self-criticism, procrastination, relationship troubles, a limited self-view, and addictions.

But there's a fourth option, and it's the one that will set you free. Rather than moving toward, against, or away, consider not moving at all. An emotion appears, and you stop. You feel caught in its grip, and you stop. In the service of peace, harmony, and well-being, you stop moving your attention into the old habits that only bring suffering. You stop creating stories that make feelings stick. You dedicate yourself to sanity, and you lovingly open your heart to what is present, as it is. The lump of sadness in your chest? Welcome it like a friend knocking on your door. The fire of anger? Let it burn if it wants to. Don't be mean to your own experience by pushing it away. Your mind may swirl, trying to convince you why you need to avoid your feelings. But don't believe it. Have courage for the truth, a longing for freedom. [6]

Here are some additional words from Rev. Keating on the subject of fear:

When fear arises, the proper response is to drop it as fast as possible, either by renewing acts of trust or just by ignoring it in your body. If we just sit through it and lap it up and say "Welcome", God comes to us in the storm. If I just wait out the storm, the presence of God will appear and the troubled waters will become calm. Fear then as an emotion, IS NOT US. When we say, "I'm afraid," this is NOT true. We should say, "I have feelings of fear". Once this distinction gets clear in your mind, you realize that feelings CAN change. The REAL you is the great "I am", the center of our being. We don't identify with evil inclinations by carrying them out. We don't project them on others and say, "They made me afraid", or, "they made me angry". We realize we have feelings, but we are NOT our feelings, and hence God can change them once we become willing. We have to tell God often, even when we're not sure it's true, "I am, willing that you take away my faults." This is much more realistic than to roll up our sleeves and say, "Well, I'm never going to be angry again". No chance". In centering prayer, we have a saying, "No thought is worth thinking about." One of the things that is very helpful in the process of healing the unconscious, is to see that we ARE NOT IDENTIFIED WITH OUR THOUGHTS OR FEELINGS, OR OUR BODIES FOR THAT MATTER. We have bodies. We have feelings. We have thoughts. But if you know you're not them, and don't identify with them, you can change them. This insight relativizes the domination they have over most people, who have not yet begun the healing process of self-knowledge. This term in the Christian tradition, is basically the exposure to the contents of our unconscious, as a result of deep rest and trust in God, and what we call contemplative prayer".[7]

What about those times when the body does act out in ungodly or unloving ways, and does things I really didn't want it to do? Well, it happened to the Apostle Paul all the time. Here's an amazing scripture truth below:

> *And if I do what I do not want to do, I agree that the law is good. As it is, it is no longer I myself (new man) who does it, but it is sin (old man) living in me.* (Romans 7:16-17)

When my being does things that I didn't want it to do, it wasn't I/new man *(Soul, Mind, Spirit)* who did it, it was the old man *(flesh)* who did it. (Ephesians 4:22). So, BE GENTLE ON YOURSELF! This is a very freeing, healing and liberating truth to many believers and wisdom seekers, who have been trapped for years in the strongholds of guilt and fear. But, this scripture truth above can also be very dangerous if placed in the hands of an untrained/uneducated person. Listen to what scripture says:

> *You, my brothers and sisters, were called to be **free**. But do not use your freedom to indulge the flesh; rather, serve one another humbly in love. For the entire law is fulfilled in keeping this one command: "Love your neighbor as yourself."* (Galatians 5:13-14)

Based on this scripture passage above, while freeing and healing it is, I know I have to be very cautious. Because, when faced with thoughts that tempt my being to engage in behaviors that are pleasurable to my senses, but negatively impact my well-being, the 'flesh' or remnants of the 'old man' identity might say:

*Hey John, just go ahead and engage in that (*fill in the blank) *behavior, for after all, it's not you who will be doing it.*

I think you see what I mean when I say this scripture truth is very healing and liberating, yet at the same time, can be very dangerous.

7

Careful Bible reading

Over time, I learned that the Bible is not easy and light reading. It's full of parables and often difficult-to-interpret passages. Placed in the hands of an untrained/inexperienced reader, like I was at one time, it can cause a lot more harm than good. I'm not saying that people shouldn't read the Bible, what I am saying is that one should be cautious and careful not to take every verse of the Bible literally. I know I'll receive many emails on this, but, it's just my personal belief based on my own personal experience and the research we've done at **Healing Info Ministries**.

The earliest Latin interpretation of the Gospels, suggests that readers not take the Bible literally. Yes, the Bible is the inspired Word of God, but one ought not take each word or phrase literally. Why? A recently discovered fourth-century commentary written by the African-born Italian bishop, Fortunatianus of Aquileia, actually interprets the Gospels as a series of allegories, instead of a literal history. I've experienced and have I've witnessed, how verses such as *'be perfect as your heavenly Father is perfect'*, and other verses, if taken literally or out of context, can bring much unnecessary guilt and suffering. Therefore, I keep the following Biblical 'themes' in mind, when reading sacred scripture:

- There is nothing that can ever separate me from God's love.
- There's nothing I can ever do to earn the eternal life of my Soul. It's a free gift.
- As a child of God, I'm equal to every other person in God's eyes.
- I'll never be able to fully understand why things have, are, or will happen the way they do. I walk by faith, not by sight.
- Restoration is and will happen, in God's way and in God's timing.
- God does mysteriously cause all things to work together for my good.

So how should we use the Bible? Here's some advice from Rev. Richard Rohr:

- Offer a prayer for guidance from the Holy Spirit before you make your interpretation of an important text. Whether you are of the conservative or liberal persuasion, this will decenter your egoic need to make the text say what you want or need it to say. Pray as long as it takes to get to this inner intellectual freedom and detachment.
- Once you have attained some honest degree of intellectual and emotional freedom, try to move to a position of detachment from your own will and its goals, needs, and

desires. This might take some time, but without such freedom from your own control needs, you will invariably make a text say what you need and want it to say

- Then you must listen for a deeper voice than your own, which you will know because it will never shame or frighten you, but rather strengthen you, even when it is challenging you. If it is God's voice, it will take away your illusions and your violence so completely and so naturally that you can barely identify with such previous feelings! I call this God's replacement therapy. God does not ask and expect you to do anything new until God has first made it desirable and possible for you to do it. Grace cannot operate under coercion, duress, shame, or guilt. Please trust me on this.

- If the interpretation leads your true self to experience any or several fruits of the Spirit, as they are listed in Galatians 5:22-23 – love, joy, peace, patience, kindness, goodness, trustfulness, gentleness, and self-control - I think you can trust this interpretation is from the Spirit, from the deeper stream of wisdom. You can trust it even if it leads you to make a formal mistake! With such good will, you will eventually see it as a mistake - and even experience will draw you closer to divine union.

- If you sense any negative or punitive emotions like morose delight, feelings of superiority, self-satisfaction, arrogant dualistic certitude, desire for revenge, need for victory, or any spirit of dismissal or exclusion, you must trust that this is not the Jesus hermeneutic at work, but your own ego still steering the ship. Watch, especially, for any subtle feelings or righteousness or grabbing on to those taken-for-granted feelings of "I am right" and "they were wrong." It might even be a solid intellectual interpretation – but it will be spoiled by your impure use of it. Christian virtue is a combination of both action and intention, and thus an art form more than a science. This is precisely why a juridical, canonical approach to morality keeps you quite superficial.

- Finally, remember the temptation of Jesus in the desert (see Matthew). Three temptations to the misuse of power are listed – economic, religious, and political. Even Jesus must face these subtle disguises before he begins any public ministry. It is a warning to all of us. Our egoic power needs do not die easily.

8

Suffering

During a church service a few months ago, the reading was about how God disciplines those he loves. I thought, *God, can't there be another way for me now to grow spiritually? For I've certainly been through enough adversity in my life, family, career and health.* What I sensed in reply was:

> *John, even though I reside in you and own you, your finite mind will never be able to fully understand why things happen the way they do. It's called walking by faith and not by sight. Remember the story of Joseph in the Old Testament, and all the trouble and turmoil his brothers put him through? All along I was present and active in his life, and Joseph later on was able to say to his brothers: "Don't be afraid. Am I in the place of God? You intended to harm me, but God intended it for good to accomplish what is now being done, the saving of many lives. So then, don't be afraid. I will provide for you and your children. And he reassured them and spoke kindly to them"* (Genesis 50:19)

Therefore, when I encounter thoughts such as: *why me, this is suffering is just not fair, or I can't endure this adversity*, I gently and proactively with my mind self, profess the truth from Romans 8:28 that somehow, someway, God is mysteriously causing all things to work together for my good.

The following are some words of wisdom on the subject of pain and suffering from well-known author, speaker, and Pastor Rick Warren, author of *The Purpose Driven Life:*

> Your pain often reveals God's purpose for you. God never wastes a hurt! If you've gone through a hurt, he wants you to help other people going through that same hurt. He wants you to share it. **God can use the problems in your life to give you a ministry to others.** In fact, the very thing you're most ashamed of in your life and resent the most could become your greatest ministry in helping other people. Who can better help somebody going through a bankruptcy than somebody who went through a bankruptcy? Who can better help somebody struggling with an addiction than somebody who's struggled with an addiction? Who can better help somebody who's lost a child than somebody who lost a child? The very thing you hate the most in your life is what God wants to use for good in your life. Redemptive suffering is when you go through a problem or a pain for the benefit of others".[8]

I've worked for religious based organizations where the leadership behaved in very unloving ways, and I directly suffered because of it. I felt powerless and very perplexed. Why would God allow a faith-based/religious organization, to have leadership in place that acted in unloving ways?

Below, are some words from Rev. Thomas Keating on the subject of powerlessness, and how it can bring much spiritual growth and benefit, if we use the gift of our mind self to choose to allow it:

> Powerlessness is our greatest treasure. Don't try to get rid of it. Everything in us wants to get rid of it. Grace is sufficient for you, but not something you can understand. To be in too big a hurry to get over our difficulties is a mistake, because you don't know how valuable they are from God's perspective, for without them you might never be transformed as deeply and thoroughly.[9]

9

Resistance to what is

Many of us are familiar with those moments in Mary's and Jesus's lives, where they both asked God that He change the difficult situations that they found themselves in. But God chose not to change their situations or circumstances, and yet they both were given the power and peace to say: 'thy will be done'. And so can we.

I think about the 'Our Father' prayer that I learned in grade school. Many of you remember the part: *thy kingdom come, thy WILL BE DONE, on earth as it is in heaven*. It didn't dawn on me until recently, that when I recited this prayer, OF COURSE God heard and answered it. Sometimes I notice thoughts of doubt as to whether or not the current circumstances that I find myself in are God's will for me. But, I've learned that when I pray and ask God that His will be done in my life, that's pretty much a no brainer. Of course he's thrilled to answer this prayer request. As painful as things may seem at the time, His will is mysteriously being done.

Some words from Dr. Brenner on the topic of 'resisting life':

> It's our natural, awakened state to resist nothing.
> When the illusion of separation is seen through,
> there's simply the free flow of experience continually

welcoming everything. There is no threat, no fear, and no sense of a person who needs to avoid or defend. It's effortless. But add in human reactions, fears, desires, and expectations, and the world divides into the duality of inner and outer, acceptable and unacceptable—otherwise known as human suffering. If you want to know the luminous peace of your true nature, then get to know how and when you resist. What is resistance? It's an activity of the agitated mind that says a resounding, "NO!" to your present moment experience. It's a desire to cling to some experiences and push others away—a desire for things to be different than they are. Take a moment to reflect: What feelings do you resist? Where in your life do you say no to what's actually appearing? Where do you want or expect things to be different than they are? Someone wrote to me recently saying she hates the way she feels when she wakes up in the morning, with too much tension and too many worrisome thoughts. Hating your experience is resisting, and resisting is a recipe for feeling stuck. You're locked in a fight with what's happening, leaving no room for the experience itself to shift or move. Resisting energizes the experience rather than giving it the liberating space it needs to come and go without attachment. We're masters at resisting our experience. How do you resist? Here are some possibilities: compulsive behaviors such as overeating, excessive use of alcohol or drugs, excessive shopping, texting, or gossiping, being too busy or preoccupied to be present with your experience, recycling thoughts of worry, judgment, complaining, or blame, resenting how you feel, or waiting for or hoping that things will change. The common motive behind all of these behaviors is to keep you from relaxing with your present moment experience. How can you possibly know the peace of your true nature if your own experience is an enemy? What's the alternative? You make the sacred choice to stop the outward momentum, slow things down, and lovingly turn inward. Things now have space to shift as you create a new and loving relationship with what arises. Instead of hating what's happening, you're friendly, open, and curious. You let things be as they are. You become the welcoming presence that ends the inner war with your experience. Why not try it out so you know how it feels? Simply go inward and say a warm and loving hello to any thoughts, feelings, or physical sensations that are present. Breathe and stay… The mind quiets as the one who wants to resist starts to fall away. With no attention to the story in your thoughts, you're one with what appears, loving it with a warm embrace like a long-lost child coming home.[10]

I strive to follow these words of wisdom from Dr. Brenner. For when I do, I experience much less stress and dis-ease.

10

Counseling

I resisted the thought of going to a counselor. For after all, I was a man. I didn't need help. I could handle everything myself. I was strong and tough. Going to a 'shrink' would be a sure sign of weakness. What would my family members, friends, or co-workers think if they found out that I was going to a counselor? I remember my cardiologist saying in a book that he had written: *"if there is one takeaway that I'd like you to take from this book, it's **don't go through your suffering journey alone"**. Well, I gave in, and looking back I'm glad that I did. As I sat in the counseling center's office waiting room one day, I happened to read a testimony from Anne Beilor, founder of Auntie Anne's pretzels. Anne talked about how counseling helped her recover from her own mental health condition. She inspired me to continue on with my psychotherapy treatment. I encourage you to read her story at: www. auntieannebeiler.com/annes-story It's a very powerful, inspiring and encouraging story.

I believe a major problem in society right now, is how to make mental health counseling more available to those who need it, but can't afford it. It is a real and serious problem. If you feel you need or could benefit from counseling, but can't afford it, I suggest you reach out to your local NAMI organization in your area, and ask them who in the area offers the most affordable counseling. In the county where I live in, we are fortunate to have one agency that provides free mental health counseling for those who meet their established criteria. But as I discovered and researched, this is definitely not the norm. We need more places like this, if we ever truly want to reach and help those with mental illness.

11

Medical care

There are a variety of medical conditions that can contribute to the development of poor mental health. I happen to have hyperactive adrenal glands. I can control them pretty good with medication. So, as part of one's healing and restoration journey, I encourage individuals to start with their primary doctor. I found through my primary doctor and associated specialists, effective treatment plans that helped place me on the right path towards better physical health.

And what about taking medication? I hated and despised taking medication. And, I had met and known of many others who despised taking medication as well. What helped me come to the conclusion that it was okay to take medication, was when I came across some writings by well-known Christian TV personality, musician, and author Sheila Walsh. If you or your loved one are dealing with a mental health issue, I encourage you to do an Internet search on Sheila Walsh. You'll find some very inspiring and motivating words of wisdom and encouragement from Sheila.

Some research studies have shown that people who suffer from chronic anxiety and/or depression, also suffer from low levels of magnesium. There's a very interesting book on the topic/subject of magnesium. The book is called *The Magnesium Miracle.* It was written by Dr. Carolyn Dean. This is something you might want to consider researching or speaking with your doctor about. I take a highly absorbable form of magnesium and it definitely helps me stay more calm, focused and relaxed. I've had chronic muscle tension since I was a young child. A relaxed body definitely helps promote a relaxed mind.

How about over use of the Internet researching health issues? I had to trust God that He would give me the necessary and needed knowledge and insight that was necessary, as long as I kept my life in proper balance. I can't recommend enough the benefit of turning off all electronic and screen devices, 2-3 hours before bedtime, if you care about your health. Research shows that excessive use of smart phones and other electronic devices, DOES increase adrenal hormone production. And having an overabundance of adrenal hormones such as cortisol in the bloodstream, does contribute to the development of sleep difficulties, medical illnesses and other diseases. I know it's hard, but, isn't your health worth the effort?

And another suggestion: unplug the power to your wireless modem and router before you go to bed each night. Why expose your body to additional electromagnetic radiation all night long, when you're trying to rest? When I started doing this, I'm convinced a saw a reduction over time in my bodily tension and fatigue.

One year ago, I was diagnosed with a leaky mitral heart valve and had to undergo open heart surgery. If one would have told me 15 years ago that I'd have to undergo open heart surgery and stay in intensive care for 10 days afterwards, my body would have very likely entered into a state of perpetual panic attack mode. But, I gently applied God's Word to the regular, normal, typical fears initiated by the remnants of the old man/flesh, and remained calm, cool, and relaxed before, during, and after the procedure. Pretty miraculous actually.

I've personally discovered that caffeine and sugar increase my anxiety levels. As far as supplements, I use Garden of Life Organic Raw Meal powder, flaxseed oil capsules, a highly absorbable form of magnesium, a multivitamin, vitamin C, and I drink tart cherry juice for its proven anti-inflammatory and anti-oxidative properties. I do believe it's a wise idea to limit the use of alcohol, based on my experiences with drinking alcohol and anxiety.

12

Sense living

Every day, I continue practicing placing my 'mind self' attention, on present moment living (*what I see, hear, feel, touch, etc.*). It's amazing how often I notice my mind self's attention is SET on thoughts that are in the past or the future. Whenever I notice I'm beginning to feel anxious, I stop and check to see where my 'mind self's' attention is focused or centered on. And sure enough, it's usually focused on some ruminating story from the past or a worry about the future. When I gently use my 'mind self' to bring its attention back into the present moment, the anxiety subsides. I do this by focusing on what I'm seeing (*clouds, cars, grass, trees*), what I'm hearing (*people, birds, my breathing, planes, trains, and automobiles*), what I'm smelling, and what I'm touching or feeling. As I said, if you're like me, you'll be amazed at how much your life has been lived with your 'mind self' set on thoughts about the past or future, rather than on the joy, miracle, and beauty of the present moment.

13

Relaxation

I learned that a relaxed body minimizes the development of anxiety. Whenever my body is tense or feeling anxious, that increases the likelihood of my brain kicking-in with its 'what if' scenarios and fearful thought and belief patterns of thinking. These thoughts and beliefs trigger my adrenal glands to start producing stress hormones, which in the past, wreaked havoc with my body. I highly recommend that if you're serious about addressing anxiety, that you engage in listening to a body relaxation audio or video. Over time, you'll notice a decrease in your body tension levels and anxiety.

As previously mentioned, I strive to listen to Dr. Gail Brenner's 'Ease and Relaxation' audio once in the morning and once in the evening. It's only 17 minutes long and is one of the best investments I've ever made for my overall health and well-being.

Another thing I learned, is the need to SLOW down. To slow down in just about everything I do. I was astonished to find myself always doing things in a rush or in a hurry. I didn't realize it at the time, but this constant rushing was causing my adrenal glands to pump more and more adrenaline, cortisol, and norepinephrine into my bloodstream. And stress hormones do what they were designed to do best: trigger fear and anxiety in the body for a perceived 'fight or flight' situation. So, I made the conscious decision to slow down in everything I did. This reduced the production of these hormones in my body, which lowered the levels of anxiety that I felt and experienced.

14

Accepting thyself

N ot knowing or understanding scripture truth, or because of some bad teaching that I might have received, I believed condemning thoughts about myself. This caused me a lot of unnecessary suffering. I'm thankful to have learned that unhealthy and/or unloving thoughts do not stem from me, 'new man/spirit' identity that I am. They stem from the remnants of the 'old man/flesh' identity that I was. They are a normal every day experience of all human beings. Listen to what the Apostle Paul said:

> *So I find this law at work:* **although I want to do good, evil is right there with me***. For in my inner being I delight in God's law; but I see another law at work in me, waging war against the law of my mind and making me a prisoner of the law of sin at work within me* (Romans 7:21-23).

If the greatest follower of Jesus that ever lived, experienced unhealthy/unloving thoughts and desires, hey, I'm in very good company. Paul was okay. I'm okay. No more beating myself up.

I love the scripture passage that says: *there's no condemnation for those who are in Christ Jesus* (Romans 8:1). I still recall this truth several times each day. Have thoughts about causing harm to yourself or others? Well guess what . . . . they're just <u>normal</u> thought remnants of your 'old man/flesh' identity, which as a Christian believer, is NO LONGER YOUR IDENTITY! Hooray!

Below are some thoughts from Rev. Keating on the need for each of us to use our 'mind self' to accept ourselves lovingly and unconditionally, as children of God, especially when the 'old man' throws flaming arrows of personal condemnation at us.

> Take and accept yourself just as you are, where you are. If you are aggressive, lustful, fearful, or shy and passive, notice your feelings before, during, and after each incident, without emotional reactions of blame, shame, anger or discouragement. Let God work with your faults and limitations. Just recognize them and be with them, without trying to correct them directly. As you watch them, feel them, and accept them, their force and exaggeration will gradually diminish. Keep moving to the center of your being, where divine love is, and be present to and welcome whatever bodily feeling or emotion that is happening. The present moment contains all we need to be happy.[11]

St. Therese said that growth in our spiritual lives is a gradual life-long process, and that it's okay that we have the imperfections and remnants of the 'old man' present. She said:

> I am simply resigned to see myself imperfect, and in this, I find my joy.[12]

15

Truths that restore

The only way of breaking the power of lies, is
knowing and speaking God's Truth
Judith MacNutt – Co-founder Christian Healing Ministries

There were many times when I felt completely hopeless, that I would one day be set free from the deep, dark recesses of anxiety that I was experiencing. By not using my mind's full capabilities to 'hold thoughts captive' as scripture instructed me to do, I was being adversely impacted both mentally and physically.

World renowned Christian healer and co-founder of Christian Healing Ministries in Jacksonville, Florida, Judith MacNutt, states above that at some point in our lives, we're to begin using our God gifted 'mind self' and 'Spirit Truth', to break the power of lies and BE SET FREE. For me, I discovered Judith was 100% spot on accurate. It was 'the way' God *redeemed my life from the pit and crowned it with love and compassion.*

St. Bernard, Doctor of the church, realized that concupiscence is not an easy thing to deal with, especially if we solely rely on ourselves. He said we **must utilize God's Word** for strength and restoration. He said:

If you attempt on your own strength, it will be as though you were trying to stop the raging of a torrent river, or to make the Jordan run backwards. What can you do then? You MUST SEEK THE WORD. You have need of strength, and not simply strength, but strength drawn from above.[13]

Listed below are some key scripture truths that my 'mind self' recalls and reflects on, when it becomes aware of unhealthy, unloving, negative or fearful thoughts:

- Nothing can ever separate me from God's love.
- God will never leave or forsake me.
- God is providing for all my needs according to His wisdom and riches.
- God is my being, dwelling within me. God has purchased and owns me.
- God does take all the normal/common/typical fears that the remnants of the 'old man/flesh self' throws my way, when I make a conscious act to give them to him.
- My present sufferings are not worth comparing with the glory that will be revealed to me day.
- I trust in and acknowledge God, knowing that he is making straight my paths.
- Greater is the God living within me, than he that is in the world.
- God is causing ALL things to work together for my good.
- Since God is for me, who cares who's against me?

- When I ask God to remove a 'thorn in my flesh', and he chooses not to do so, His grace is sufficient for me, for His power is being perfected in me.
- When my body does something I did not want it to do, it wasn't 'Me' (*new man*) that did it, it was the '*old man*' that did it.
- God IS restoring me and making me strong, firm, established and steadfast.
- God's Word is setting me free.
- When people mistreat me unfairly and I end up suffering because of it, for some reason like Joseph in the Old Testament, God will bring good out of it.
- When I come to Jesus weary and burdened, in silence, solitude, and stillness, I'm mysteriously nourished, strengthened, and renewed by His doing.
- I have the strength for all things in God, who gives me the power.
- I give thanks in all circumstances.
- I live 'by faith' in God's Word and not by what I see happening around me.
- Although I want to do good all the time, like the Apostle Paul, the desire to do the things I don't want to do is right there with me. So, not only am I **gentle on myself, I'm gentle on others as well**, because they too experience the same struggle.

16

Love

*There is no fear in love. But perfect love drives out
fear, because fear has to do with punishment*
(1 John 4:18)

There are many definitions and writings on the topic of what love is. At our ministry, **Healing Info Ministries**, we came across a reflection/teaching on the topic of love that we first shared in one of our weekly blogs a few years ago. It's from Rev. Richard Rohr, a globally recognized ecumenical teacher. He is a Franciscan priest of the New Mexico Province and founder of the Center for Action and Contemplation (CAC) in Albuquerque, New Mexico:

> God loves you precisely in your obstinate unworthiness, when you're STILL a mixture of good and bad, when you're gloriously in flux. You're not a perfectly loving person, and God still loves you totally. When you participate in that mystery of being loved, even as the mixed bag that you are, you can receive the gift of forgiveness. And as far as I'm concerned, that's the only magnetic center that

knows how to forgive other people, especially when people have really screwed you, really betrayed you, really humiliated you. And sooner or later, this happens to all of us. When I can stand under the waterfall of infinite mercy and know that I am loved precisely in my unworthiness, then I can easily pass along mercy to you. God cannot *not* see his son Jesus in you. You are the body of Christ. No amount of effort will make God love you any more than God loves you right now. And despite your best efforts to be terrible, you can't make God love you any less than God loves you right now. To sum it all up, I do not believe there is any wrath in God whatsoever - it's theologically impossible when God is Trinity. [14]

What comforting, healing, renewing, transforming words from Rev. Rohr to remind me that there is **nothing in the entire universe and in all of God's creation, that can ever separate me from God's love.** And there's nothing I can ever do to earn it. It's a free gift. I simply choose to desire it and accept it. God's loving presence is right here, and always has been. Here are some words from the Psalmist:

> Where can I go from your Spirit?
> Where can I flee from your presence?
> If I go up to the heavens, you are there;
> if I make my bed in the depths, you are there.

If I rise on the wings of the dawn,
if I settle on the far side of the sea,
even there your hand will guide me,
your right hand will hold me fast.
If I say, "Surely the darkness will hide me
and the light become night around me,"
even the darkness will not be dark to you;
the night will shine like the day,
for darkness is as light to you.
(Psalm 139:7-12)

17

Forgiveness

Forgiveness is probably the greatest healer there is. In the story of Jesus, the ultimate act of forgiveness comes near the end, when Jesus says from the cross, "Father, forgive them, for they know not what they do.". Now, if you can forgive someone for torturing you and hanging you on a cross, you can forgive anything. And why forgive? Because they know not what they do. This forgiveness comes from a deep spiritual understanding of the causes of suffering – and also of those who inflict suffering, for those who inflict suffering have always had suffering inflicted upon them at some prior time. When we start to realize this, our heart opens. I'm sure you've seen images of the sacred heart of Jesus – that big red heart in the middle of Jesus' chest radiating forgiveness to all of humanity. It's one of the most potent symbols of the whole Christian tradition. It's Jesus' greatest gift, the most powerful healing balm that exists. (Adyashanti)[15]

As Adyashanti states above, the image of the Sacred Heart of Jesus is one of the most potent symbols of the whole Christian tradition. When I spend time in silence, stillness, and solitude, I have right next to me, an image of the Sacred Heart of

Jesus. It reminds me of the fire of God's love and the blood of His mercy for 'ME'.

Forgiveness, for whatever reason, is one of the hardest things for me to do. I can only ask the Holy Spirit for help. The remnants of the 'flesh/old man' self still conjure up strong feelings or emotions of hatred and anger toward those who have wronged me or who have treated me unfairly. Things are coming around slowly but surely. Just typing this paragraph is bringing up thoughts and feelings of anger towards those who've wrong wronged me, especially in my career and professional life. I still have to use my mind self's full capabilities by taking a few deep breaths, acknowledging and holding the angry thought captive, and proclaiming like Jesus did: *I forgive them, for they knew not what they were doing.* I know this is the right thing to do. Not just because Jesus did it, but because as mentioned in Chapter 6, since the people who wronged me may have not wanted to wrong me, then it wasn't really them that did it, it was the sin living in them that did it. Pretty eye opening and humbling isn't it?

18

Cast that care

'Cast your cares on the Lord and he will sustain you; he will never let the righteous be shaken' (Psalm 59:22).

'Cast all your anxiety on him because he cares for you' (1 Peter 5:7).

Most of us have read or have heard these scripture verses numerous times in our lives. But how many of us actually make the conscious effort to regularly apply them each day? I know I don't.

Now, after I handle anxious thoughts, feelings or emotions in an appropriate/healthy manner, I believe God still wants me to 'cast' or 'give' Him the anxiety. In the beginning when I first started doing this, I really didn't notice much of a decrease in my body's anxiety levels. I learned that's totally normal. My adrenal glands were just in the 'habit' of injecting stress hormones into my bloodstream. But in time, the fearful feelings did lessen and they rarely occur now. I learned that for me, there was no better advice that I could receive, on how to handle anxiety and fear, than to follow these words from the Apostle Peter above.

I remember listening to Joyce Meyer one day talk about her

life transition from an anxious/stressful one, to one of trusting and resting in the Lord. She said something to the fact: "*for a long time it seemed like all I was doing all day long, was casting this and casting that care on the Lord.*" A great testimony from a very spiritual and gifted individual who has touched the lives of thousands, if not millions.

I'm still slowly dying to the 'flesh/old man' self each and every day. God's Word promises me that He will sustain me.

19

God's presence

"What prevents us from finding happiness? It's a lack of the sense of the presence of God. We feel alienated from God, so the world is a frightening place. If we had the sense of union with God, we'd not be afraid. But since we do not, we feel alone".[16]

"I keep my eyes always on the Lord. With him at my right hand, I will not be shaken" (Psalm 16:8).

What prevents us from finding happiness? It's a lack of the sense of the presence of God. These words from Rev. Keating and the Psalmist above, remind me of my need to consciously remember throughout each day, that God is present 24/7. As mentioned by Rev. Keating above, the 'old man/flesh' will try to get me to believe that God has abandoned me. or that I'm all alone. But brother and sister, remember this biblical truth: *'greater is the God that lives within us, than he that lives in the world'* (1 John 4:4). As the Psalmist says above, the Holy Spirit, our helper, who we are the temples of, will help us keep our eyes fixed on the Lord so we aren't shaken. I just love the scripture Truth below that says:

God has said, **never will I leave you never will I forsake you.**

So we say with confidence, the Lord is my helper; I will not be afraid. What can mere mortals do to me? (Hebrews 13:5-6)

I remember during my 40's, there was a time when I experienced so much fear in my being, and God felt so far away and distant, that I carried around in my work shirt pocket an image of the Sacred Heart of Jesus to help **remind me** of God's infinite love, mercy, and presence. In fact, I placed next to my bed a vintage chalkware piece of the Sacred Heart of Jesus that I purchased on eBay. It, along with thousands of others, were produced in the 1950's and 60's by Michigan Composition and Lamp Company, a company founded by Joseph Giuliani, and a place where his daughter Nancy Viviani worked. Nancy passed in 2017. I never met Nancy, but my heart and Spirit has a strong sense of admiration for her and her family. I've actually purchased several of their Sacred Heart of Jesus chalkware pieces from the 1950's and have given them to people who were experiencing anxiety, or a feeling that God was not present or had abandoned them. Some people wear jewelry, some get tattoos, and others take other actions to remind them of God's omnipresence. That's good. Find whatever works best for you.

I purchased and wear a necklace with the symbol of the Eternal Knot on it. Every time I put it on or take it off, I'm reminded of the indwelling presence of the Holy Trinity in my being. Just one more aide or tool in my journey from fear to faith.

Happiness is union with God. There is no place without God. Whatever you do, you should feel that it is God's work. God is acting through your body. He is thinking through your mind. He is working through your hands. [17]

There is no greater meditation than the constant remembrance of God at all places and at all times. When you practice this, you will lack nothing and will be ever blissful. [18]

20

Peace

Many people will say that the most important spiritual goal in their life, is to be able to find inner peace. Well, one can easily find hundreds of opinions and definitions, as to what the word 'peace' actually means.

The **Healing Info Ministries** team discovered one particular definition of the word 'peace', that we felt was quite powerful and descriptive. While I was experiencing my 'Dark Night of the Soul' experience, I held fast to this definition. It brought me much comfort and consolation during the most difficult times and moments. It's taken from the writings of William Barclay, Scottish author, radio and television presenter, Church of Scotland minister, and Professor of Divinity and Biblical Criticism at the University of Glasgow:

> Peace is that tranquility of the heart, which derives from the all-pervading consciousness that our times are in the hands of God.[19]

Our times are in God's hands. When it's all said and done, I, new man (*Soul, Mind, and Spirit*), believe by faith, that **my time is in God's hands**. It is a surrendering of my entire being to the God who owns me, who created me, and with whom my Soul will joyfully live forever with one day.

Here are some very powerful words of wisdom from Dr. Brenner on how to love our emotions and thus experience more peace:

Don't be attached to always wanting peace and happiness. When emotions visit you, don't avoid them. Because you'll be missing out on an opportunity for melting barriers inside you. Being with emotions is simple, once you get the hang of it. It's just about letting the energy run through you.

- First you notice the emotion: You'll say, "I'm angry," or you'll become aware of a wave of upset or unhappiness.
- Take a breath and pay attention to the sensations as you breathe.
- Then turn toward the emotion, and hold it in the wide-open space of being loving and aware. Let the sensations in your body be. Welcome the energy or power or agitation or numbness.

When your attention gets drawn into your mind and you're grabbed by a lot of thinking, gently bring attention back to your body and breath. Don't wish for your experience to be any different than it is. Just breathe, open, and let things be.

And when you welcome the emotion fully, you'll feel it. You

might sob or scream as it moves through, and this is okay. It's being released and liberated. Be with your emotion like this for as long as it feels right—maybe 30 seconds or a half hour or more. You'll know. *You're just flowing to the next thing.* When strong emotions arise, they can be overpowering. They occupy your mind so you can't focus on anything else. If you're panicky, deeply feeling grief, or in a rage, you might find it too hard to relax and let the emotions be. Maybe they feel out of control and too strong. This is when you take a different approach that honors the emotion but gives you some space from it.

- Take several deep breaths, filling your lungs in the front, side, back, top, and bottom…then exhale.
- Soothe yourself physically by hugging yourself or stroking your arm or shoulder. As you do this, focus your attention on the sensations.
- Put your hand on your heart or belly. Take a few breaths.
- Try this grounding practice. Put your attention on the situation you are in and name what you're perceiving. For example, go into nature and say, "the air on my skin, the birds chirping, trees moving in the wind."
- And another grounding practice. Stand up and feel your feet on the earth. Feel grounded right where you are. Then breathe or name things or put your hand on your belly or heart.
- Reflect on what you really want for yourself in the moment, and say "peace, calm, relaxation, steadiness." Repeat whatever words resonate for you like a prayer.

Once you're not so overwhelmed, turn toward the emotion directly and let it in like the loved one that it is. It will untangle naturally when it's met with love and acceptance.

Emotions run through you, but they're not you. Let them come and go, and here you are—awake and alive in this very moment.

21

The restoration promise

"And the God of all grace, who called you to his eternal glory in Christ, after you have suffered a little while, will himself restore you and make you strong, firm and steadfast. (1 Peter 5:10)

This Truth above, became a powerful mainstay for me. It's a very liberating biblical truth, that still comforts me to this day. God will restore in his way and in His timing. But the truth remains: **GOD WILL RESTORE.** This is why I believe the Apostle Paul, even in the midst of his sufferings, was able to attain a state of peace and contentment. He knew by faith in the Word, that his restoration in God's way and in God's timing, would happen. A wonderful joyful promise that each one of us can hold onto as well.

22

Healthy life-style tips and resources

Walking is man's best medicine
Hippocrates

I know there are thousands of books out there on the subject of health and wellness. Based on our research, we found one book in particular titled *The Whole Health Life,* written by author Shannon Harvey, that we thought deserved extra special attention. The book covers a wide range of thoroughly researched healthy lifestyle topics, such as stress, emotions, food, sleep, healthcare and relationships. We think you'll enjoy it as well.

The **Grace Alliance** is a not-for-profit organization that cultivates healthy solutions for hearts and minds through simple, innovative biblical truths, scientific research and practical tools. You can visit their website at: **mentalhealthgracealliance.org**

Kay Warren is the co-founder of Saddleback Church. Kay is an international speaker, best-selling author, and Bible teacher who has a passion for inspiring and motivating others to make a difference with their lives. Kay is also a board member of the National Action Alliance for Suicide Prevention. When her youngest son Matthew took his life in April 2013, her life was dramatically altered by the catastrophic loss. As she and her family continue to grieve the loss of Matthew, she became determined to be a voice for those living with mental illness. Her message to the faith community is to eliminate stigma, shame, and fear and to create warm and accepting places of refuge for those who suffer. Visit **kaywarren.com/mentalhealth/** for some excellent biblically based mental health resources.

NAMI, the National Alliance on Mental Illness, is the nation's largest grassroots mental health organization, dedicated to building better lives for the millions of Americans affected by mental illness. Visit **nami.org.**

23

The key Truth

I f there is one takeaway that I'd like you to take from this short
book about my personal and professional work experiences
with fear, worry and anxiety, it's this short prayer below that I
wrote. It has become my guiding mantra or motto, when I notice
an unhealthy fearful thought bringing disturbance to my being. I
still G-E-N-T-L-Y use it several times each day. It has been a 'life-
saver' for me, literally:

> *Jesus, I acknowledge, accept and welcome this normal fear*
> *generated by the remnants of the old man/flesh, who I (Soul &*
> *mind) used to be united with to form my former/false identity.*
> *But now, having received the Holy Spirit, I (Soul & Mind &*
> *Spirit) are united with 'You', to form my new/true identity.*
> *So, we don't worry about life, the body, or tomorrow.*

Keep watching for John Patrick's upcoming books in his Christian Mental Health series:

Depression, Despair and Hopelessness
Temptation, Addiction and Dependence
Anger, Resentment and Envy
Guilt, Forgiveness and Mercy

For more information on the subject of healing, visit the **Healing Info Ministries** web site at: www.healinginfo.org

To contact **Healing Info Ministries**, you can email: info@healinginfo.org

Endnotes

1 *The Cloud of the Unknowing & the Book of Privy Counseling.* Huston Smith and William Johnston. Image books. Doubleday. 1973. pg. 81.

2 https://www.merriam-webster.com/dictionary/soul

3 https://en.wikipedia.org/wiki/Concupiscence

4 *The Great Themes of Scripture – New Testament.* Richard Rohr and Joseph Martos. St. Anthony Messenger Press. Cincinnati, Ohio. 1987. Pages 89-90.

5 *Dark night of the Soul by Saint John of the Cross. Doctor of the Church.* Third revised edition translated and edited, with an introduction by E. Allison Peers from the critical edition of p. Silverio de Santa Teresa, C.D..

6 www.gailbrenner.com

7 *Divine Therapy and Addiction – Centering Prayer and the Twelve Steps.* Rev. Thomas Keating. Lantern Books. March 2011, Pages 84-85.

* www.gailbrenner.com

8 Crosswalk.com. Your Pain Often Reveals God's Purpose - Daily Hope with Rick Warren - November 7, 2016.

9 Contemplative Outreach newsletter. June, 2014.

* *What do we do with the Bible?* Richard Rohr. CAC Publishing. Albuquerque, NM. 2018. Pages 52-54.

10 www.gailbrenner.com

11 Contemplative Outreach newsletter. June 2015

12 *Therese of Lisieux. Story of a Soul.* Chapter VII. Page 158.

13 *Bernard of Clairvaux. On the Song of Songs.* Volume IV. Sermon 85. Number 1,4. Pages 196-97,200.

14 *The Divine Dance and your transformation.* Richard Rohr with Mike Morrell. Whitaker House. New Kensington, PA. 2015.

15 *Resurrecting Jesus –Embodying the Spirit of a Revolutionary Mystic.* Adyashanti. Sounds True Inc. Boulder, CO. 2014. Pages 90-91.

16 Contemplative Outreach newsletter. Rev. Thomas Keating.

17 http://www.saibaba.ws/articles2/all_that_remains_is_my_sai.htm
18 https://sathyasai.us/devotion/discourse/manifest-divine-within-you
19 *The Letters to the Galatians and Ephesians.* William Barclay. Revised edition. Westminster Press. 1976. Page 50.